ACADEMY METHOD

A

DANCER'S DIET

By
Ken Ludden

This book is intended as a textbook companion to the Academy Method
Instructor Certification Program and should not be used for any other
purpose.

First published by Lulu, May 1, 2013
ISBN: 978-1-300-99743-6
Printed in the United States of America

TABLE OF CONTENTS

Chapter 1 - A Dancer's Body

Nearly everybody has said, or heard someone say, "I wish I had a dancer's body." Indeed, a dancer's body is an ideal. It is strong, flexible and beautiful to see. It moves with grace and has a posture of dignity. When a dancer enters a room, it is as though they are walking on air, are bigger than life, and have a kind of confidence envied by most. But more important than all of that put together is the fact that it is achievable by anyone.

For anyone who is out overweight and out of shape, it may seem impossible to achieve, but that is not true. To achieve a dancer's body requires just two things: 1) exercise, and 2) diet. Ironically, these are the same two things that all weight loss programs require. Of the two, exercise is almost more important than diet, only because if a person begins to exercise regularly, they will soon crave other foods, more water, and begin to steer away from fatty foods just because of the way the body feels after eating them.

Exercise

For many, repetitive exercise is too boring to face every day. It takes a very special person to get up early every day and swim, run, lift weights, do aerobics, spin, power walk, jog, do yoga or do calisthenics. But when a person takes a dance class, no matter what style of dancing, they find that the exercise in dancing is satisfying, exhilarating and seems incredibly purposeful. The variety of step combinations and routines in dance is infinite, and so one can never be bored. But on the opposite side, working on a piece of choreography, making it better and better, refining and polishing it, never get tedious because there is always purpose in the movement. The better the movement becomes, the more one feels its sense of purpose. In fact, once a person starts dancing, they almost always become dedicated to it, for the greater degree of control one has, and the more technical ability, the more expressive the movement becomes. And there is nothing more fulfilling than to have truly expressed one's self.

The exercise in dance also is beautiful, powerful, inspiring and compelling. To feel in command of the body is a very good feeling, and to express what you feel is also a good feeling. To do these while integrating music with the body is pure joy. And to do all of these and know it looks great to others is an amazing feeling. So when considering a diet, knowing that exercise is essential for the diet to truly be effective and its effects lasting, turning to dance is the only logical solution.

ENDORPHINS AND MOOD

Once a person starts to become active, the activity causes the body to release endorphins into the blood stream. This instantly elevates mood. Many people who are overweight and out of shape are also suffering from some degree of depression. Though most likely not clinical depression, the depressed feeling of sedentary life is a self-perpetuating trap. It is hard to get out of bed, or off of the couch, and electronic media can distract the mind from the fact that the body is not being used.

Try watching movies or playing video games for many hours without snacking. It is very hard to do. Most snack foods are fatty, salty, or sweet and each of these by itself makes the body feel lethargic. So the longer you sit, the more you snack, and the more you snack the longer you sit. The next thing you know getting showered and dressed is easy to put off, and before you know it you are living in PJs or sweats!

EXERCISE AND SLEEP

At the end of the day, without having exercised, it becomes harder and harder to feel tired and to sleep soundly. And so eating a heavy meal, or intense snacks, before sleeping helps you fall asleep. But you wake up hung over from sugar or fat. Salt makes the heart race, and that alone can make falling asleep, or sleeping soundly, more difficult.

The effect on mood, then, when exercise is introduced is extreme by contrast. And many people get so exhilarated by exercise that they over do it the first day or first week, get an injury (or become very sore) and then settle right back on the couch, chips and soda in hand.

Considering everything, dance class is the perfect exercise for getting in shape, or losing weight. The best news is that if you pursue it, in the end you will have a dancer's body.

BODY CONSCIOUSNESS

Beyond the aspects of diet having to do with extreme or unusual circumstances for the individual, all dancers must develop a unique awareness of and communication with their body. When a child first starts studying dancing it is important that all foods that have noticeable, unnatural, temporary or pacifying effects on the body be removed. This of course means soft drinks, artificial food substitutes (artificial sweetener, petroleum based vinegars, additives even if nutritional, colors, flavor enhancers, etc.), but it also means particular foods or food derivatives that boost circulation, relaxation, quick impact on blood sugar levels, and nutrition-based psychological supports even when they are natural and healthy foods.

VASCULAR SYSTEM

Things such as wheat grass, ginger, and ginseng are all natural but they artificially boost the heart rate, increase circulation, alter the vascular system, and effect mood. Likewise, hot milk before bed, celebrating by overeating, giving food rewards and the like are quite normal, but must go. There are many ways to help someone sleep (reading a story, singing a lullaby, massage, soaking in a warm bath, etc.) that do not create associations between food and states of mind. Using the eating of an piece of fresh fruit, or any other natural food source or derivative, to give a sudden energy burst is misleading to the communication between awareness and the body. And employing any sort of binge-purge mechanisms to maintain or alter weight is very dangerous in young children.

RULES FOR MAINTAINING DANCER'S REGIMEN

The reason for these rules is not that a dance student's life is to be miserable at all. In fact, establishing many ways of dealing with life's guaranteed requirements (sleep, fatigue, hunger, over excitement, adrenalin bursts, falling in love, feeling competitive, etc.) should be met with as much celebration, preventative or supportive preparation, acknowledgment and fun as possible. The reason to do it with anything other than food is for a very specific reason. When a regular diet is maintained, with good balanced meals, calm and enjoyable atmosphere around eating, healthy and ample snacks, fresh foods, and all other dictary positives, the dancer is able to grow properly and advance in an ultimate way. Part of this development, which happens quickly if nutritional distractions and falsifications aren't introduced is that the dancer will develop a close and reliable consciousness of what the body needs and when it needs it.

YOUR GENIUS BODY

With pet puppies it is recommended to place the same amount of food, at the same times in the day, out for the dog to eat very consistently. At the end of the day if there is food left, throw it away. This way the dog will learn to eat as much as it needs, depending on how much exercise it is getting. This works to some degree with other animals as well, but it is most effective with dogs. All mammals have this instinctual ability, including humans. There are some differences of course, and one of them is that humans eat a much wider variety of foods.

In our society we have learned this lesson for humans, but only with females and pregnancy. There are many jokes about the strange dietary cravings of expectant mothers, but there is a very good reason for allowing the mother to eat precisely what she wants, as much as she wants, when she wants it. As the fetus develops, different parts of it develop. The type of nutrients needed to build a brain are quite different from those needed for lungs, bones, muscles, blood, heart tissue or skin. The mother has an intimate communication with her body and her developing child, and knows through this instinct what she needs to eat.

To be raised in your dance life with a consistent balanced diet, the dancer will find an equally intimate communication with their body, and will experience cravings much like a pregnant woman. It is important to know what is in the foods that are craved, so that healthy and additive-free sources can be found. Craving pickles or grapefruit, for example, is indicative of needing potassium; craving pretzels or chips is indicative of needing salt.

Once this is established it must be maintained. Even, and especially, when a dancer retires and for the remainder of life. For being able to give your body exactly what it needs will keep a dancer from becoming enormously fat upon retirement and the loss of constant exercise, and it also guarantees maximum health, which increases in importance as age advances. And so, for every dancer who is active in their dancing career, there are differences in the dietary approach that renders the best results.

CHAPTER 2 – A DANCER'S DIET

Along with exercise it is necessary to eat right. Over the centuries dancers have learned that there are different maximal diets for different segments of their lives as dancers. This book is organized do address the dietary needs of each segment. These segments are:

1) Training,
2) Performance,
3) Travel, and
4) Days Off.

Each phase of a dancer's life requires different dietary considerations. To develop a dancer's body, whether you are a dancer or not, is an exciting thing. This book will show you how. But first, can you do this if you are not a dancer? Yes you can!

A DANCER'S DIET FOR THE NON-DANCER

If you are not a dancer, you will find that the same segments exist in the life of every person. At the beginning of each section of this book, we will point out how the segments relate to parts of general life. Each section, then, gives examples of matching phases of activity for the non-professional dancer. This way you will know exactly which phase of exercising you are in, and therefore which type of diet is appropriate.

MORE THAN DIET AND EXERCISE

But there is more to consider than how diet joins with exercise. You also have to think about resting, stretching, sleeping, grooming and personal hygiene, because they all come into play.

To dedicate yourself to a new way of living, so that the diet will not only make changes in your body but also in your life. It is important to look at what you do when you are not eating or exercising as well. We've already talked about how exercise effects mood, and then how mood effects sleep, energy level, willingness to work, and appetite.

Most people are aware of the need to "cool down" after intense exercise. But what about after the "cool down" period? What do you do when you get back home and have piles of laundry to deal with, a dwelling to clean, bills to pay, a social life to maintain, and relationships? If the new you is going to be around for a long time, then everything else in your life becomes related to this.

You will have to learn how you feel at different points in the day, when to rest, when to stretch, when to do chores, and how to live with your new dancer's body and all it takes to keep it.

NEW WAY OF LIFE

Each segment of exercise requires different dietary patterns, and often this means that mealtime will be at a different time than usual. It may mean you need to nap, or stretch, or go shopping for supplies in a different pattern than what is usual. It is important to make your life support this new you, and that means getting others to understand, and be thrilled about, what you are doing, why you are doing it, and how.

Dance is perfect for this, too, because it is a performed art form, and you will eventually have public performances they can come to, even if it is just a studio showcase. And before long you will probably find some of your friends and family who want to do it to. There's nothing better than that kind of active support.

In the end, if you follow this book, you will have a dancer's body, and a new lifestyle. You will find a new joy in life, and more energy than you may have felt before.

So, on to the diets!

DIETS

Each person's system is different, and there is no perfect diet for all people. For dancers, in particular, it is essential to know one's body precisely. Allergies are usually obvious, and there need be no explanation of why one must avoid allergic reactions.

More difficult to pinpoint is a truly maximized result, when the near maximum may appear exceptional, and certainly better than before. A subtle lack of energy will often go unnoticed when the adrenalin of performance is upon you. There is an extreme periodic fatigue dancers naturally experience due to a workout that will often mask symptoms of dietary-induced fatigue.

A dancer must be fully aware of the body and its needs at all times. Like everything else about dancing, it is a very special and very impressive life. And since "you are what you eat" it is very important to be allowed to develop and maintain a body consciousness associated with diet.

WHAT CLASS LEVEL IS PERFECT FOR YOU?

Exercise in dance class is divided into levels: beginning, intermediate and advanced. And no matter what the levels are called, nor how many tiers there are within a level, taking class at your level is not likely to cause you to overdo it. And to know your proper level you must rely on an experienced and highly qualified teacher.

With aerobics class, spinning, running and free weights there is a far greater risk of overdoing it, and many instructors are more drill sergeants than qualified instructors, so they may not notice when something is too much for and individual in the class.

SEGMENTS OF A DANCER'S LIFE

Below is an analysis of the different life segments every dancer will endure, and what is happening in the body at the time. Some suggestions will be made as to how to meet the needs, counter the effects, and be best prepared for the demands. But remember that every single individual is different and unique. It is vitally important that dietary options be explored (under supervision) and any anomaly be taken seriously. In the end, each dancer must know what his or her body needs, and provide it – in advance.

SEGMENT 1: TRAINING

When a dancer is in training, several elements are most certainly involved. The body is being trained in order to develop muscles (or new uses of muscles). Each element places specific stress on the system, and these stresses must be prepared for, balanced by and effectively supported by dietary adjustments. Below are the various predictable elements, how they impact the body, and what dietary balancing is most effective. However, each dancer is unique and so must remain very attentive to what the body desires in terms of foods. Adjustments must then be made, beyond the material listed below, so that the body gets what it needs.

TRAINING SEGMENT FOR NON-DANCERS

For a non-dancer, even one who is taking dance class as a means of exercise, it is important to know when the activity in your life qualifies as a Training Segment for the body. The catch phrase is: when you are first learning or practicing new movements.

ACTION PACKED VACATIONS

These times might include getting ready to go on vacation that will include skiing, swimming, surfing, hiking, horse back riding, hang gliding, wind surfing, open air festival dancing, etc. Any time you will be doing physical movements that are not the norm for your daily routine you will need to prepare the body in advance.

TEMPORARY CHORES

When you are helping someone move, doing estate inventory when someone has died, baby sitting for a newborn or toddler, video taping an event, attending a book sale, stuffing envelopes, setting up tables for a wedding, visiting a museum or castle, or spring cleaning, you are going to be doing movements with your body that are not the norm for you. This will involve new muscles.

LIFE CHANGES

When you get a new job, change modes of transportation in your commute, become pregnant, or start a new hobby that will be ongoing in your life, you must prepare the body for the new use of muscles, joints and coordination. Even moving to a different office, if it comes with a new chair, different level of drawers in your desk or new direction for reaching the phone, keyboard, reference materials, etc., all of these will demand new muscle combinations and must be prepared for.

Pregnancy is a very important life change. Everything about it is new, even if it isn't your first child. And this requires a training segment diet as well as nutrition for pregnancy.[1]

NEW MUSCLE GROWTH AND USE

Each of the above represent a different example of Training Segments in life. Training involves simultaneous development of new or augmented musculature and intense familiarity with new types of coordination, balances, positions, rhythms and specific communications with the audience. Each new development must first go through a phase of preparatory exercises designed to build the appropriate muscles, and/or inculcation of new interrelationships of movement/expression elements. All of this is accomplished through repetition, and most rapidly assimilated into reflex knowledge

---

[1] If you are pregnant and taking dance classes, doing yoga, martial arts or any other rigorous activity, find experts in both pregnancy and the sport or activity. It may take a team, but in the end you will sail through without injury and with maximum growth and development. For pregnancy information, teachers of the Bradley Method of childbirth are among the most qualified in terms of diet and pregnancy while active.

when that repetition is progressively pushed to the point of exhaustion.

TRAINING SEGMENT NUTRITION

This combination of factors calls for a high protein diet, rife with fibrous sources of carbohydrates and periodical availability of sources of quick energy.

The period of exercise sets up the need in the body for the growth that will occur after exercise is initiated. Most muscle growth occurs in the hours after the exercise period, however it begins while that period is in action.

Therefore, nutrients that will be used by the body to form the new muscles (or to enhance existing muscles, provide energy fuel so extant muscles can adapt to new combinations of muscle use and timings) must be in the body and broken down into essential elements so it is ready to be absorbed or put to use.

ESSENTIAL ELEMENTS OF NUTRITION

There are three basic such essential elements: mineral components (such as calcium), proteins and glucose. Mineral components are used to strengthen bone density, provide elasticity to tendons, and other such jobs in the body. Proteins are used to build new muscle fibers, or enhance the development of new ones. Glucose is the basic fuel the body burns as its energy source to do everything it does, including thinking.

To have these essential elements in the body, broken down so that they will be available for immediate absorption requires a diet that provides particular elements at particular times.

BODY FUEL

The first thing the body will use in the exercise session is the fuel, or glucose. Glucose is closely related to fructose, the natural sugar found in fruits. Therefore to consume fruits early in the day, and perhaps as a snack during the day, gives the body an immediate supply of glucose.

But this glucose comes in relatively small amounts from fruit, and is mixed with a high concentration of water in the fruit itself, and so both the time it is in the system and the amounts provided are small.

TIMING OF MEALS

When one eats the large meal in the middle of the day, or soon after exercise, contains large amounts of carbohydrates, these will be digested and turned into a store of glucose during the night and following morning, and so provide a constant supply of glucose for the exercise period. Remember, that thinking also is fueled by glucose, and the more the body has, the more it can use for energy and to focus and take in new ideas and other learned elements.

TRAINING BREAKFAST – GRAIN-RICH

A good solid breakfast is not advisable for dancers if it contains starches and large amounts of protein. However, an egg (or egg white) is good along with a balance of grains[2] and fruit is the best way to start the morning. Including grains for breakfast is very important because it gives the body fiber.

This breakfast is specifically designed for the training segment of exercise. But it is also good on a regular basis. The way the body takes in and processes food, turning it into usable fuel, is the same no matter what you are doing. Yet when training, there is

---

[2] This awakens the digestive system, which starts the body breaking down the carbohydrates and proteins from the previous day, but also will start the digestive system working. In fact, for people who need to lose wait through dieting, eating grains for breakfast will greatly improve weight loss because it starts the digestive system first thing in the morning every day.

new muscle development to worry about, and this is the main basis for this meal.

Repetition

During training periods when a dancer is learning something new, and throughout the process of training the body to do movements automatically, repetition is one of the most powerful and successful tools. Yet when the body goes through a period when a particular movement, style or position is repeated at the exclusion of other things (as is often the case), the body is having an unbalanced demand made of it. There is no way around this temporary, but common, situation. To remove intensive focus or repetition from the method would result in half-learned, compromised, or misunderstood steps and sequences. The dancer, without this repetition, would also apply what was usual rather than truly embrace what is new, different and specific of what is being learned.

And so, repetition is a given in classical dance training. This being the case, there are predictable results, and preventable problems. To explore these, it must be understood what some of the challenges are in such a period of time.

Below is a table that shows which foods contain high concentrations of these essential minerals.

MINERAL	FOODS WITH HIGH CONTENT
SODIUM	Sodium and chloride are the elements that form common table salt. Canned vegetables; prepared salads, such as potato, macaroni or egg salad; snack foods, including potato chips, crackers and corn chips; prepared soups, sauces and condiments all contain sodium. Processed meats, such as ham, hotdogs and beef jerky offer high levels of sodium. Of course, table salt is also a good source of sodium and chloride.
CALCIUM	Dairy products, including fresh milk, cheeses, yogurt and ice cream, all have high levels of calcium. Spinach, kale, bok choy, Swiss chard, and turnip, collard and mustard greens and other leafy green vegetables all provide calcium. Other fruits and vegetables that contain calcium are broccoli, oranges, green beans, dried beans of all types, mushrooms, asparagus and cabbage. Salmon and sardines with the bones intact and oysters are also good for adding calcium to the diet. Tofu, prepared with calcium chloride, is also high in this electrolyte.
MAGNESIUM	Grain products top the list of food items that deliver the electrolyte magnesium. Breakfast cereals in particular are often fortified with magnesium. Other plant-based sources include leafy green vegetables, dried beans, bananas, apricots, cashews, almonds and peanuts. Both tea and coffee are good sources of magnesium. Brazil nuts, which grow in magnesium-rich soil, also offer good amounts of the mineral.
POTASSIUM	Try oranges, peaches, nectarines, pears, bananas and melons. Dried plums are particularly high in potassium. Other sources include beans, both fresh and dried, spinach, squash and brussels sprouts. Meats and fish also provide dietary potassium. Many salt substitutes use potassium chloride instead of sodium chloride.

The first is that the muscles, or muscle groups, being exclusively used will get overworked. This is part of the design, and there is nothing wrong with it (see the next section "Exhaustion" in this chapter). As a result, the muscles that are over-worked will become depleted of sodium, calcium, potassium and magnesium. Together, these are called "electrolytes." The depletion of these electrolytes in the muscles will cause cramps anytime from during the training session to within the next 72 hours unless sodium, calcium, magnesium, and potassium are replenished. It is possible to avoid these cramps through diet and dietary supplements. A diet rich with these minerals is the very best preventative against muscle cramps.

TRAINING LUNCH - MINERAL-RICH

The intake of minerals should be done in the middle of the day, such as having a salad with spinach (iron) and a light cheese such as cottage cheese, feta or some other goat-milk cheese, or pine nuts (all calcium rich foods) along with tomatoes, carrots, asparagus and other vegetables rich with minerals.

TRAINING SNACKS – MINERAL-RICH

Mineral-rich foods make excellent snacks throughout the day. Most of these foods contain both minerals and vitamins. And the body holds stores of minerals and vitamins that it will dip into as needed throughout the day. Having a constant replenishing of these nutrients through the day is very good.

TRAINING DINNER - PROTEIN-RICH

Proteins come from foods such as eggs, meats, fish, and dairy products. There is protein in some nuts as well. Protein-rich foods often digest slowly and tax the system a great deal. During the rehearsal day it is not a good idea to eat any heavy proteins, because the body energy will be pulled in two directions—to fuel digestion, and to provide energy for dancing. Therefore, during a period of training, it is best to eat a meal containing proteins after the active part of the day is finished.

Having a steak, omelets or other such protein-rich dishes for the evening meal, or supper, is advisable.

Vegetarians and Protein

For those on a vegetarian diet, it is important to be sure that you are getting a complete protein. For example, a meal that includes protein from beans must be balanced by a starch (such as rice, tortillas, potatoes, or another grain such as barley, or quinoa), and also a secondary source of protein such as cheese. Beans contain protein and carbohydrate, but by themselves do not comprise a complete protein. Make sure that with your protein you also take fiber, to assist in breaking the protein down in digestion.

SEGMENT 2: PERFORMANCE DIET

During performance periods many things in the daily life of a dancer must shift, some things must change. The body needs to be at peek performance in the evening, between 8:00 pm and 11:00 pm during the week, but then in the early afternoon as well as night for matinee performance days. Some companies change their company class time for performances, making it later in the day, and some do not and leave it at 10:00 am. Regardless of the time of company class, it is during performance that the dancer must be at peek.

TIMING OF MEALS CHANGES

This means that the timing of food, sleep and other dance related parts of life must shift to later so that the dancer's biorhythms and habitual cycles can shift to be aligned with the new timing and focus of each day's events. The basic diet is the same as the diet students use for optimum efficiency.

There are many changes required at performance time.[3] Often the daily class starts later in the day, or if it is at the same time it will be repeated in the early evening as a pre-performance warm-up. During Tech Week[4] dancers are often in the theater all day, and that will not necessarily be in the same location as the studios and regular dressing rooms.

You may go to sleep later and wake later in the morning. You may need to bring all the food you will eat throughout the day with you, or spend extra money at restaurants near the theater for mid-day meals. You will

---

[3] In European professional companies that are associated with Opera Houses, dancers perform nearly every night of the season. If they are not dancing an evening concert, then they are participating in an Operetta, Musical, or onstage in a Drama. Therefore the daily schedule is consistent throughout, and they often have a long break mid-day so theater personnel can tend to chores only done during business hours. The meal structure remains the same, however, during performances of dance concerts, while the timing remains constant.

[4] This is the week before a performance run begins. At this point the dancers know their parts, costumes and props are made and in use, and the choreography is finished. The theater technical crew, then, is hanging lights and backdrops, constructing fixed set pieces, focusing lights, having rehearsals with special effects, orchestra or sound equipment. Tech Week is hard on dancers, and often engages them for far longer hours, with far less exercise.

sometimes have to shower at the theater after a performance, or even bring a rolled foam mat to take a nap, or do prolonged stretching tucked away in some corner of the back stage or elsewhere in the theater complex.

For male dancers, it is necessary to change the timing of when you shave from morning to evening starting a week or more before the performance run begins. The body develops a cycle of facial hair growth based on habit. For about 3 or 4 hours after your normal shave time the hair on your face does not grow at all, or does not grow as fast. This is quite like the phenomenon of plants ceasing growth for a time when they have been relocated into new soil.

And for all dancers, it is necessary to alter any habitual moving of the bowels. The body will have developed a rhythm throughout the day of when it empties its waste. This adjustment should also be made a week or more prior, even if it means changing meal time, so that you do not develop cramps during a performance.

These are but some of the changes you will need to make to accommodate performance in the theater. In time, with experience, this adjustment will become like second nature. But at first, it is important to focus on your body, and train it and yourself to approach everything differently so that the performance will not be damaged or made less effective due to nutritional or personal hygiene routines.

PERFORMANCE AND NUTRITION

Overall, the very best diet for any human, particularly for physically active individuals, is to eat six to ten small meals each day, heavily packed with protean, grains, fruits, nuts and roughage. With such a diet changes in schedule are immaterial, because the routing covers waking hours uniformly. But in our culture there is a very different pattern established, and to break free of it is impossible for most people. Therefore, below is an outline for a performance diet.

PERFORMANCE BREAKFAST – GRAIN AND PROTEIN

The first meal of the day, normally called 'breakfast' should be filled with grains, some protean, and loads of vitamins. Fresh fruit with yogurt and granola is perfect, as are health shakes and or smoothies. Some people operate at their best with a substantial hot meal, but even this must contain fiber and grains (such as grits, oatmeal, farina or some other cereal).

The primary objective of the first meal of the day is to wake up the digestive system[5] and move nutrients into the blood stream. Having a good solid meal of protean gives fuel to be used in the evening during performance, but it is the grain and fiber that allows the carbohydrates and protean from the evening before to be absorbed as glucose to immediate use during warm up and rehearsals during the day.

The first meal of the day should be eaten within one hour of waking up. If one starts the day with exercise (swimming, stretching, yoga, tai chi, or some other) then the meal should be eaten just after this exercise is completed.

> NOTE: Be careful of caffeine and other stimulants. If taken into the system before a meal, then they can become a meal substitute, which is extremely bad for the body, and perhaps the very worst

---

[5] For people who are dieting, one of the best tools for losing weight is to eat breakfast. Many seek to lose weight by not eating, but when we sleep the body shuts down and digestion stops. Until it is woken up by the first meal of the day, those nutrients just sit in the system and turn to sugars.

thing a dancer can do during a performance week.

The second meal of the day, normally lunch, should be primarily salads, fruits and some light form of protein like yogurt. Here it is the chewing that is of importance. When we chew, the body floods the digestive system with fluids that break down food for absorption. By eating salad one not only is chewing, but also the fiber, minerals and chlorophyll from greens all work as instant energy for the body. Fruit, containing fructose, comes into the body readily and keeps blood sugars even and steady.

The second meal of the day should be eaten at a logical break in the activities (between class and rehearsal, or between rehearsal and stage warm up), making sure there is enough time to eat and then rest for at least a half hour. This period of rest allows the body to put all of its energy to digesting the food just eaten.

PERFORMANCE DINNER – CONQUEROR'S TRIUMPH

When dancers eat varies from dancer to dancer. In first writing this book the meals in the Performance Segment were listed as: first meal, second meal, third meal, etc. This is because during performance runs the daily life of a dancer is extremely different than during rehearsals and training. Of course the same is true for traveling and days off. And so the choice was made to stick to the normal: breakfast, lunch, dinner and snack sequence. But even that didn't quite fit.

When performing dancers experience something very few others experience. During a performance the dancer forgets their personality, their identity and fully gives themselves over to the performance at hand. There is a magic on the stage that alters reality.

Imagine the kind of focus you have when you are getting married. You are yourself, of course, but you are "being" a bride or groom And that day, everything you do leads to the wedding, or follows it with life transformed. The same is true when a baby is born, or you participate in a sports match. There are many such events in life, were described earlier in this segment.

During this time, the body is in full use and that use is intensely monitored by the individual. You are aware and actively crafting very step you take down the aisle, every action you make when the ball is in play in a sports match, and every word you speak or angle of your head during a momentous public address. This concentration is supported by the body without hesitation, without reservation.

The body must have absolute power, and a vast supply of energy. This is the fuel, the glucose, spoken of in the start of this book. And the body will keep a constant supply coming throughout the performance, often leaving you exhausted when the adrenalin wears off, and usually starving. The body has just depleted every reserve of mineral, protein, oxygen and glucose. And these must be replenished.

To do this there must be a meal in the day that is heavy with protein. Some dancers eat a thick steak, others an omelet with 6 or 8 eggs. Some will make a huge tower of a sandwich with many forms of sliced meats and cheeses. This protein feast is essential.

Professional dancers often will combine this with the post-performance late supper, and take their protein and carbohydrate together. Some will go out right after a performance and have a steak and salad, then after they are home will have a large helping of pasta as they wind down and wash out their tights, leotards and other dance apparel and hang it to dry over night. And some end the day with a big bowl of ice cream as they listen to the music they will need to interpret the following day.

This meal is so vital it cannot be under-emphasized. Without it your muscles will atrophy, and your body will start to consume your own skin to get enough protein to rebuild the muscles. If, during a performance run, you are starting to have skin troubles,[6] it is most likely because you do not have enough protein in your diet.

PERFORMANCE LATE-SUPPER – CARBOHYDRATE FEAST

The third meal, normally dinner, should be heavy in protein and carbohydrates.[7] The third meal is what will provide the energy for the following day's exercise period (class and rehearsal). It is also the meal that will provide the nutrients for rebuilding the body tissues that have been over stressed during

---

[6] Many dancers suffer from this and blame it on nerves, or the repeated use of stage make-up. When looked into, it is most often found to be a lack of protein in the diet.

[7] If there will be a forth meal, then the third meal should be heavy in proteins, with some greens, and the carbohydrates should be saved for the forth meal, after performance.

performance, or over worked due to the extreme nature of performance schedules.

SEGMENT 3: TRAVEL DIET

Dancers travel as a way of life. Often, dancers are referred to as "theater gypsies" because they must constantly travel to where the work is. Even in large companies, touring quite often brings in needed revenue for the company, and supplies the company with essential critical reviews, publicity promotions and public networking that helps the company thrive.

AIR TRAVEL

When traveling, particularly by air, it is important to keep your nutrients plentiful. Dehydration and loss of electrolytes are two major contributors to jet lag and general fatigue from travel. To counter this there are several things to do.

WATER – ETERNAL LIFE SPRING

First, be sure to drink water, but more importantly drink fluids that are full of electrolytes and their components. Orange juice, grapefruit juice or tomato juice are among the very best things to drink while on planes. And be sure if you eat food to eat natural foods (tuna fish, fruit, nuts, trail mix and the like). This will create a constant replenishment of the nutrients being lost.

But it is possible to prevent many of the circumstances that cause the depletion within the body.

JET LAG – CONSTANT COMPANION

The effects of jet lag and travel depletion are caused in part by the pressurization of the interior of the airplane, and in part by the very dry and re-circulated air within it. The increased intake of fluids will help with the dry air effect, and bringing along some anti-viral tissues can protect against some airborne viruses.

The effect of pressurization is impossible to escape, though it can be lessened. When the interior of the aircraft is pressurized it places stresses on the body, and the best defense the body has is to be able to respond to changes in pressure by equalization of the pressure. Any tight or restrictive garment will not allow the body to equalize evenly, causing stress. It is helpful to loosen belts and any restrictive clothing. However, the clothing is not the main culprit—shoes are.

When the shoes are kept on during a flight, the body responds to pressurization unevenly. The best way to adjust to this is by taking off your shoes, and wearing loose fitting socks. It is important to follow a simple rule:

> Take shoes off while still on the ground, and put them on again when you are back on the ground.

This way the entire body can equalize the pressurization evenly and organically. The effects of jet lag and travel depletion will be minimized.

The final culprit is the lack of sleep. Most sleep lost on airplanes is not because of the subtle movements of the airplane, but because of the sound of the air rushing past the outside of the plane. Wearing earplugs will greatly help with sleeping on the plane.

TRAVEL BY GROUND

When traveling by ground, there are a variety of means by which companies get around. Each way of traveling brings its own reality. Each has down sides to proper nutrition, and offers opportunities as well. The most important thing is to know precisely what sort of travel will be demanded of you, and to prepare well in advance so that you have everything you require.

BY AUTO

Travel by automobile means you will be in a privately owned vehicle, or a rented or leased one. Either way you will have authority over the vehicle and only be restricted as to what you can carry with you by the amount of room available. You will also have control over when and where the vehicle stops.

Research your route and find out what restaurants and shopping establishments are along the way. Talk to the driver and find out when you will be traveling, and then check those times against the different retail outlets you may need to use. Remember that restaurants in cities are open far longer hours than those in less populated areas. And don't count on having 24-hour pizza or deli delivery when you are on tour. Regional habits are vastly different from one place to the next.

Also find out if the foods you normally eat are available, and what they cost. Organic foods are unheard of in some places, or outrageously over priced. Local areas will have certain foods that they produce, which means lower cost and higher quality, and others that they must import, which means the opposite.

Bring along plenty of non-perishable snack foods, but be aware if traveling far from home if there are any restrictions at border crossings.[8] Bring what you need, that you are allowed to bring, and then find out what substitutes for prohibited items will be found when you arrive.

When traveling it is very easy to become ill in reaction to new climates, pollens, water, foods and elevations above sea level. Nothing is worse than traveling to dance, teach or learn choreography and becoming ill and missing out on the experience.

In a car you also can bring a small stove or cooler with you. This can keep you close to your normal diet and absent of the rigors of adjustment to foreign foods.

In a private automobile you will have limited space, and it is often impossible to stretch out. Bring a pillow that is comfortable

---

[8] Islands have major restrictions on plants and soil organisms being brought into their environments. Places like Australia, New Zeeland, Ireland, and Indonesia have very strict rules, because the introduction of certain foreign elements can cause blight, disease, drought or livestock catastrophe. Also in the US, some states have border crossing restrictions. California is one such state.

to you, and some sort of cover (blanket, sheet, shawl, etc.) to cover yourself in case of a draft.

Find ways to stretch out, do not wear restrictive clothing, and have easily removable shoes. It is hard to get relaxed and comfortable on a long journey, and you will find that muscles cramp and joints get sluggish and sore.

The blood vessels in your body are muscles, and when they are in a fixed position for a long period of time, they become cramped into position. If you suddenly get up and move around after an extremely long trip, it is possible to get little ruptures in the blood vessels, and there is danger of thromboses. Be sure you stop and stretch.

As for the shoes, it is very common to remove your shoes when on a long trip in a car. But with the twisting, turning, bending and flexing of your body, and the constant flow of items inside of the car, shoes can become lost or hard to find. Be organized in the space available, and when you take off your shoes, find a place to put them where they will be likely to remain, and from where they can be easily retrieved on rest stop.

By Bus

When dancers travel in a bus or a van, they have far less control over the route, and will not necessarily have more room for luggage since the space is shared. Find out what the reality of the travel will be and plan for it.

In the bus and truck tours of the mid- to late-20th century, companies often traveled in busses without bathroom facilities, and then were restricted by union or administrative limits as to when, where and how often they would stop. If you are in such a situation, eat very little before you get on, and keep liquids to a minimum. There is nothing worse than the distress of being prevented from going to the bathroom while driving, or the humiliation at having to go in the woods at the side of a roadway. Plan ahead!

On the itinerary of most bus tours there will be planned stops at restaurants and rest stops along the way. Find out where they are, and what foods are available. You want to stay as familiar as you can to what you normally eat.

You also need to stop and stretch. Remember, like in a car, you will be in a relatively limited, fixed position with not much range of motion available, and your muscles will cramp, your circulation will be inhibited and your joints will become compacted in your lower spine.

By Train

Trains have café cars, and some have proper restaurant cars. This is excellent, and quite convenient when there is a restaurant, but the quality and selection of foods can be limited. Café cars notoriously have terrible food in a train, and the types of snacks available on the aisle carts that some rail services maintain are mostly sugar, starch and fat.

Find out if there is a dining car, and if so their menu will likely be published and available to the general public. Do your research and your preparation.

If traveling for a long period by train, get a cabin, or sleeper space if you can. Otherwise, if on trains with individual cabinets in which 6 or 8 people can sit in two rows facing each other, choose a seat mate. This way you can sit opposite each other and put your feet up on the seat opposite.

Trains allow you to get up and walk around. Do this, and stretch. You will arrive much more relaxed and have much more energy.

TOUR

When on tour it is essential to carry with you healthy snacks. Try to eat familiar foods, and stick to the many small meals plan as best as you can. Remember that foreign foods will cause the body to react in unpredictable ways.

TOUR BREAKFAST

Tour breakfast is an institution. In the United States it is traditional to stop at Denny's. This is a restaurant chain that serves good breakfasts. On tour you will find you want a hot breakfast, with some protein (egg, sausage or bacon) and then some sort of grain.

Birchermuesli (more modernly called "muesli") is a combination of rolled oats and nuts and berries mixed with yogurt. It is quite common around the world and gives all of the elements you need, except it is not hot. It will do, but it is good to have some toasted, grain-rich bread that is hot along with it.

TOUR LUNCH

Lunch on tour is normally found at a restaurant, and for dancers a nutrient packed salad works best. A Cob, Waldorf, Caesar, or couscous salad will give the variety of ingredients needed to keep the body going, hydrated and energized without slowing it for an energy depleting digestive process.

Alternately a moderate and light sandwich can give the dancer the correct balance of nutrition, hydration, minerals and proteins. The difficulty is finding what is needed in the variety of locales one faces on tour.

If you are in a foreign country, be very careful of fresh fruits, salads, raw foods and water. All of the fresh foods will have been rinsed in local water, and that water can make you very sick.

In the end, tour lunch is quite safely replaced by tour snacks. This assures you have control over what is entering your body, and you can protect against being exposed to local water.

TOUR SNACKS

When on tour, snacks are your most important meal. The human body is designed to do best when 6 -10 small means are eaten each day. Each meal consisting of mainly grains, nuts and fruits, with occasional protein. During the day bread, or some other form of carbohydrate, is continuously consumed in small quantities; and also legumes, in the form of leafy greens, are to be munched throughout the day. This gives the body the variety of nutrients at intervals, and keeps the body operating at its maximum.

On tour it is wise for dancers to eat in this way, and carry in the dance bag a wide variety of nutritious snacks that will constitute, across an entire day, complete nutrition. It is also true that raw foods are easier for the body to digest and absorb. Many snack foods are in raw form, or have been dried without first being cooked (freeze-drying is a method that imitates this badly, but is better than nothing).

With your tour snacks, however, you must make sure that there is ample fluid, and for this tomato juice or orange juice are the top choices because they contain electrolytes.

TOUR DINNER

When on tour, be certain there is a restaurant that will be open after you are finished with the performance, and the post-performance things that will take your time (greeting members of the audience, removing make-up, and coordinating with management for following day adjustments to schedule.

If you are able to find a restaurant that is open, a good solid protein and carbohydrate meal is the proper thing to eat. If you are unable to find anything other than a pizza place open late, then get pizza with extra cheese, and a thick crust. Of course pile on the toppings you love, for a dancer's body knows what it needs.

If your tour takes you to a place without public eateries open late enough to serve post-performance meals, then you must plan ahead. During the day buy yourself a solid protein and carbohydrate meal, and feast in your hotel room.

SEGMENT 4: DAY-OFF DIET

As previously stated, rest is an essential part of every dancer's regimen. One should take one day each week without dancing. This allows for all of the development gained during the active days prior to be assimilated. It also is able to prepare for the next week's work.

It is also important to schedule vacation time. Your body will need to rest, and for the dancer, resting is an art form. Below are the elements of rest that make it constructive, enjoyable and essential for the dancer to maintain their body while on vacation.

4 Rs of Rest

On this day off it is important to recuperate, refresh, replenish and rebuild. These '4 Rs of Rest' are accomplished in activity as well as in diet. Each of these elements is discussed below specifically, but you will see that there is quite a bit of overlap between them in terms of diet and nutrition.

Vacation Breakfast: Recuperate

The morning of a day off the muscles need to have a break in their routine. Massage and a relaxing stretch session are good ways to begin that day. There will be excesses of toxin expelled from the muscles into the lymph system, and it will need to be urged on its way through the body filters and out as waste. Drinking liquids (such as cranberry, lemon, lime, melon, and various teas that stimulate the kidneys and bladder) that flush the system help in this process.

The night before a day off eat a large meal with complex protein (steak, lobster, pork, etc.) and follow it with more heavy proteins with breakfast (bacon, ham, sausage, eggs, cheeses, etc.). This will give the body an entire day to break down and absorb these without body energy being directed toward muscle work.

This regimen for the morning of a day off will help the body recuperate from any damage done. Swimming and leisurely strolling is very good for a day off, so long as it is done as recreation and not exercise.

VACATION SNACK: REFRESH

On a day off it is important to have an outing, explore something new and interesting, do something exciting you've always wanted to do, and to try new foods. If sushi is a rare treat, go for sushi. Likewise, if there is a new recipe you want to try, a new food product that is being talked about (sometimes there are exotic fruits and vegetables on the market), or a food you've heard of but have never had, this is the time to try it.

By introducing something new to the diet it wakes up your taste buds, and stimulates your digestive process. Just be sure this new item isn't junk food or something manufactured with dietary toxins or complicated chemicals. You want to refresh your system with something new and different, yet that still provides good nutrients. There also is a lot to be said for different combinations of foods, because they work together in the system in slightly different ways. A day off is a perfect time for trying something new.

VACATION LUNCH: REPLENISH

In the middle of the day eat lots of salad vegetables, grains and nuts. This packs the system with minerals, but also the fiber stimulates the digestion so that the heavier proteins eaten earlier are broken down. Add pepper to these foods, because pepper also stimulates digestion.

VACATION DINNER: REBUILD

In the early evening eat a large meal of carbohydrate, and then a very light salad to end the meal. This will ease you back into your normal routine and prepare you for returning to work.

CHAPTER 3 – A DANCER'S INJURIES

DEALING WITH CRAMPS THROUGH DIET

If a dancer has cramps, or is entering into a training period (learning new choreography, taking a master class intensive series, etc.) and anticipates that muscles might be worked in such a way that cramps will result, diet alone may not prevent it. In this case, Dolomite[9] is an excellent supplement as both preventative and anecdotal remedy. Dolomite is a natural substance that contains calcium and magnesium fused together by nature. It has been found that when dolomite is mined and taken as a supplement, the proportions of the two minerals are so perfectly balanced that the body absorbs it all.

In the late 1970s there was a problem with one manufacturer of dolomite, and one of the veins of the mineral deposit had traces of lead in it. In reaction to news of this consumers stopped buying dolomite.

---

[9] One can find dolomite, and it is important to find "mined" dolomite, rather than artificially compiled dolomite. It remains the very best natural supplement, and the company Nature's Plus still sells natural, mined dolomite tablets.

Distributors, whose products were fine and beneficial, sought to reassure the public by creating a new form of dolomite in which calcium and magnesium were separated out of the source ore, purified, and then re-blended. This artificially created dolomite was then promoted widely.

The problem with the artificial dolomite was that very little of the minerals were absorbed by the body. It is not clear what was extracted in the purification process, but whatever it was, the result was that people were consuming a mineral supplement that gave them no benefit whatsoever. Due to this production of dolomite stopped for the most part.

There is an old myth, perpetrated by a misunderstanding of some scientific discoveries at the dawn of the 20th century. Scientists saw that when the muscles became overworked they produced a derivative of Lactic Acid called Lactate.[10] Since sore muscles often occur the day after an intense workout, and at the time of muscle activity Lactate is produced, they assumed that

---

[10] Lactate is identical to Lactic Acid, with one fewer protons, so it is for all intent and purpose the same, yet it is important to call things by their correct names.

muscle soreness came from the presence of this acid, and that Lactate is responsible for muscle fatigue. More recent science has discovered that the opposite is true.

Muscles use oxygen for fuel when they are working. When muscles are worked intensely, they use all available oxygen stored in the blood, because they are using it more quickly than the oxygen breathed in can be delivered. The body responds first by switching absorption methods, so that instead of relying on the oxygen stored in the blood, it starts using the oxygen that is being breathed in directly, bypassing the storage stage. This moment is called "getting a second wind" by runners, triathlon competitors and players of other endurance sports. The type of exercise that uses oxygen directly as it is breathed is called aerobic.

But when the body is pushed yet further, it begins a type of exercise called hyper-aerobic.[11] And this is when the body starts producing lactate. Lactate is a substance that fuels the muscles without oxygen. It is what

---

[11] In class structuring, the hyper-aerobic exercise portion (prolonged petit allegro, extreme repetitions of jumps, long passages of continuous motion, etc.) should optimally be 8.5% of a training session.

allows the body to keep going without muscle fatigue.

The body can do more, however, and in training must be pushed beyond the hyper-aerobic to the super hyper-aerobic[12] state. This type of exercise demands of the body to produce an excess of lactate, because what is being produced is being depleted more quickly than it is being produced. This is the next "second wind" endurance athletes refer to, and is accompanied by a flush of hormones that cause slight euphoria. In this state, lactate is produced not only in the muscles, but in the tissue immediately surrounding them, and after the workout is what makes the muscles seem enlarged for some time. In fact, it was the detection of this excess store of lactate that led to the myth that it was responsible for muscle soreness the day after an intense session.

Science now has discovered that 100% of the lactate produced by super hyper-aerobic exercise is absorbed by the body within four hours of ending your session.

---

[12] Also discussed in the discourse on class structuring later in this book, the super hyper-aerobic type of exercise should never exceed 5% of a training session.

So, what causes the muscle soreness? It isn't known for certain, but most likely it is due to the micro-tears in the muscle fiber discussed earlier in this chapter in the section on Muscle Bulk.

EXHAUSTION

Applying the principles of movement as they relate to classical theatrical dancing allows the dancer to make use of all elements of motion with absolute efficiency, to the maximum degree appropriate, in order to achieve artistic communication with the audience. Each of these goals is trained into each dancer. Yet absolute efficiency of movement is not something a dancer learns to do. It is achieved by the absence of effort; the allowance without obstacle of all relevant forces. It is what the dancer does not do that achieves efficiency.

When the body is exhausted, utterly exhausted, yet is demanded to perform a movement, it will override the obstacles of mind, diminished energy supply and resistant circumstance. The body itself, independent of the dancer, will perform at absolute efficiency.

Therefore, exhaustion is carefully designed into training so as to achieve this goal. A dancer who is pushed into super hyper-aerobic exercise through repetition and careful sequencing of muscle uses and coordination will achieve absolute efficiency. And just to have gotten to this point also means that the movement becomes automatic, therefore is performed naturally as well.

Given that exhaustion is an intentional part of the plan in training, the body will respond as all bodies do to the state of exhaustion. The dancer must, therefore, have stores of nutrients in their diet that can be converted into lactate. This nutritional balance comes from all of the dietary elements discussed thus far in this section.

DEHYDRATION

With exhaustion comes sweating, and having been pushed to the furthest edge, the dancer will have sweated enough to become dehydrated. Remember, when the body feels thirst, it is already dehydrated. Every dancer must drink not only water, but also liquids that provide electrolytes and nutrients, and have a water supply close by during sessions, though not in a way that disrupts training sessions.

Should a dancer become seriously dehydrated, it is very important to replenish the body with all that is lost, particularly sodium. Athletic fluids are designed specifically for this purpose. Drinks such as Smart Water and Gatorade are good, but not meant to replace a balanced diet.

ELEMENTS OF NORMAL ROUTINE ELIMINATED

Also true of the body in training is that the normal routine is skewed for the purpose of making time for, and concentrating focus on, the new material being learned. Adjustments to accommodate those new additions to the routine have already been covered. There is another issue, however, that will also require adjustment to dietary intake.

Dancers, from intermediate level on, know well the specific issues they must continually work on, and each has a routine followed with the loyalty of the superstitious. In addition, every dancer has things they enjoy, parts of dancing the use to indulge themselves, or parts of the body they feel requires constant focus or their entire ability to dance will suffer, perhaps critically. During times of training, particularly when new movements or new choreography is being learned, there is little or no time for these. Dedicated dancers will find a way to include these elements of their routines, and due to the young age of dancers, normally do this by cutting out both food and sleep.

Injuries increase, learning of the new material slows and becomes inaccurate, and focus diminishes. Lack of sleep results in more frequent feelings of hunger, and cravings for "quick fix" types of food sources become common. Increased stress will temporarily erode relationships and place even more stress on the dancer in all areas of their life. Fresh fruits and raw vegetables for snacks, fruit juices and tomato juice for hydration, and easily digested foods (such as sushi, soups and stews, dinner salads or omelets) are the best basic elements for a dancers diet in such circumstances. And at such times, protein rich shakes are recommended rather than instead of steaks and other heavy, slowly digested proteins.

Youthful arrogance, along with the Peter Pan syndrome common in dancers, dictates that they will most likely ignore instructions, particularly in times of stress. Therefore it is extremely critical that good nutrition be an automatic part of each dancer's routine from the youngest age.

CHAPTER 4 – A DANCER'S RECIPES

Dancers are very tuned in to the needs of their bodies, much like pregnant women. They will crave the sort of foods that will deliver the particular nutrients needed by the body. But this is not the case for students until the very end of their training. In this chapter is a collection of recipes that various dance professionals, or those who know them well, have put together for the different segments of their career.

TRAINING RECIPES

During training you want to have an efficient use of your energy throughout the day. Having foods prepared in advance allows you to use your energy where you need to, rather than in the kitchen. These recipes are all easy to make, and for the ones that must be prepared just before you eat them, they are simple and quick, leaving a minimum of dirty dishes to wash.

BREAKFAST SHAKE

(Sallie Wilson)

This is an effective way to start the day, and will improve your system. Even you hair will have a healthier glow to it when you eat this shake during training.

Ingredients:

3 eggs

1 banana

1 tblsp. Peanut butter

1 tsp. vanilla

2 tsp. Brewer's Yeast[13] (de-bittered, powder)

2 tblsp. Wheat germ

1 tsp. bee pollen

1 tsp. Agave nectar

2 cups milk

4 ice cubes

Put all in blender, and mix at high speed until thick and smooth. Be sure that ice cubes are completely broken down, this assures that everything is mixed well and gives a frothy texture.

This will carry you throughout the day without hunger, and provides plenty of protein as well. Ingredients can vary to taste, but be sure that you have the same mixture of minerals, protein, liquid and fructose.

---

[13] The reason this is a peanut butter and banana shake is that those flavors go together to match the flavor of the yeast, which some people find offensive.

Breakfast Fruit Tart

(BQ)

This recipe was given to me by Hilda "BQ" Hookham, Margot Fonteyn's mother. She said she made this for Margot when she was a young dancer in training because it was the only way she was able to get little Peggy to eat fresh fruit.

It is an excellent and delicious snack, and also serves as a good quick breakfast food. It can be kept refrigerated for up to one week, is served cold, and can be made with any sort of fruit or berry that is preferred. This recipe is enough for two 9" pie tins, or a half sheet baking dish (13" x 18").

Pre-heat oven to 350° F.

Never-Fail Pie Crust

(Rita Ludden)

1 stick butter
1 3-oz. packet of cream cheese
1 cup sifted white flour

Place all ingredients into bowl and mix by hand until they form a single ball that does not stick to the bowl or the hands. Divide into halves. Each half is one face of a normal 9" pie tin (top or bottom). In this recipe you can make two open faced tarts in these pie tins, or one sheet.

Roll pie crust to ¼" even thickness and then place into pie tins or backing sheet. Create edge on crust.

FRUIT TART FILLING

Ingredients:

3 medium sized fruits (apple, pear, peach, etc.)

1 cup Assorted berries or grapes

1.5 cups milk

2 eggs

1 tsp vanilla

1 tblsp. Honey or Agave

Cut whole fruits in half, remove seeds, core or pit and then slice each half evenly. Arrange skin up to densely cover bottom surface of pie crust. If a fruit has particularly thick or tough skin, then think of where you will be likely to cut out servings to avoid having to fight unnecessarily with the skins. Fill in open spaces with grapes and/or berries.

Be creative and artful here, as you will certainly impress friends and guests with a gourmet-appearing tart!

Mix liquids in a mixing bowl and beat until slightly frothy but not into foam. Pour over fruit evenly and tilt dish to make sure liquid spreads evenly.

Place in oven and bake 1 hour, or until custard has risen in the center, and edges of crust are deep golden brown. You must be sure that egg custard is fully cooked.

Let sit uncovered for two or more hours, until cooled and all excess liquid has been evaporated or released as steam.

Cover with waxed paper or breathable plastic wrap and refrigerate. Once the custard is set, cut into serving sized pieces for easy, quick retrieval.

PROTEIN BARS

(Ken Ludden)

Dancers live on protein bars, usually manufactured ones. These usually have quite a lot of sugar, however, and are not good for the overall health of the dancer. It is far better to make your own.

In this recipe you will find standard proportions of ingredient "types" and baking instructions. Below the recipe is a table of alternate ingredients organized by "type" so that you can make bars that suit your taste. Be creative with this, and experiment with other ingredients as well.

Pre-heat oven to 275°; place parchment or waxed paper on bottom surface of flat, full sized cookie sheet, or prepare flat cookie sheet with oil, shortening or spray-on covering like PAM (after which it is good to place a light layer of salt, pepper, flour, poppy seeds, or other ingredient).

Ingredients:

6 cups flour [Type : base]

2 tps salt [Type : seasoning]

1 tsp cayenne [Type : seasoning]

1 cup black sesame seeds [Type: nutrient]

1 cup finely grated romano cheese [Type: nutrient]

½ cup olive oil [Type: liquid nutrient]

½ cup water [Type: liquid]

½ cup milk [Type: liquid nutrient]

4 eggs beaten [Type: liquid nutrient]

In large mixing bowl place all dry ingredients including the base, seasonings and dry nutrients. With a whisk, mix and aerate the ingredients until they are evenly mixed throughout.

In a different bowl (preferably copper) place all of the liquid ingredients, and beat until thoroughly mixed and slightly frothy.

In the large bowl with dry ingredients, create a crater in the center by pushing the ingredients to the sides. Pour the liquid mixture into the center of the crater.

With a wooden spoon, stir the liquid, gradually and evenly working in the dry ingredients on the sides. When all dry ingredients are thoroughly mixed with the liquids, turn dough onto a flour-dusted parchment on a counter top. Knead this mixture until it develops a low-sheen satin surface and holds together in a single ball without sticking to your hands.

> NOTE: sometimes it is necessary to adjust the mixture to achieve this step. If it is too wet, then add your base in small amounts until correct; if it is too dry then add water to it in small amounts until you achieve success.

Place your prepared cookie sheet next to the dough, and then begin pinching small amounts of dough and forming it into small sticks approximately the size of your little finger, and place them in neat rows on the cookie sheet being sure there is ¼" of space between them as they will slightly rise in baking.

If you have decided to have your protein bars rolled in an outer coating, then roll the finger-sized bars in that coating before placing them on the sheet.

Place in oven and bake for 3 hours, or until noticeably deep golden brown on the tops. Remove and let cool before storage. If you place them in a contained space too soon then liquid in the form of steam will make them stick together, and can cause them to mold if not eaten right away.

This recipe will yield about 120 bars. Kept in a dry place they will last just about as long as crackers last. Remember that commercially manufactured foods will not last as long as homemade ones, simply because there are many additives required to go into commercial foods. Many of these extend the shelf-life of the product, but can have undesirable effects[14] on nutrition. Eating five of these per day will give needed protein, carbohydrates and nutrients.

Dancers live on protein bars, and by making your own, you have absolute control over the nutrients that come into your system, and the flavors you will taste. You are encouraged to experiment with this recipe and insert many different ingredients.

Below is a chart of alternate ingredients you might select, but do not be limited to these. Any flavor you like can be worked into protein bars. This chart is meant to open

---

[14] See The Feingold cookbook for Hyperactive Children by Ben F. M.D.; Feingold, Helene S. Feingold and Pat Stewart (1979)

the door to possibilities, and broaden your horizons.

<u>*PROTEIN BAR INGREDIENT CHART*</u>

TYPE	OPTIONS
BASE	flour (wheat, rye, whole wheat, graham, barley, rice, semolina); corn meal; gluten-free flour; bajri flour (or kurakkan); corn flour; blue corn flour; nut flour (almond, hazelnut, cachew, etc.); chick pea flour; etc.
SEASONING	rosemary, dill weed, cardamom, savory, basil, parsley, cayenne, ground clove, nutmeg, turmeric, oregano, dried violet, herbs de Provence, marjoram, thyme, sage, cumin (seed or powdered), etc.
DRY NUTRIENT	caraway, poppy seed, dried fruit, dry grated cheeses, pine nuts, pumpkin seeds, raisins, fenugreek seeds, mustard seed, peanuts, green pepper corns, sea weed, sesame seeds, citron, rind, rolled oats, bean curd, quinoa, wheat germ, farina, couscous, etc.
LIQUID NUTRIENT	plain yogurt, cow's milk, goat milk, sheep milk, rice milk, almond milk, fruit nectars (pear, peach, pomegranate, etc.), tea (the stronger the flavor the better), whey, Tabasco sauce, mustard, wasabi, salad dressings, sesame oil, oyster sauce, plum sauce, etc.
COATING	sea salt; cracked pepper; mint leaves; orange; lemon or lime zest; paprikosh; poppy seeds; etc.

In the chart we do not include prepared spice and flavoring mixes (BBQ sauce, nacho flavoring, etc.) because many of them contain MSG. MSG is a radical free agent in the body and many people have, or develop, severe allergies to it. Being a radical free agent means it never leaves the body, and if in time you develop an allergy then you may have chronic problems you can never be free of. Be very careful when you take in such seasonings as MSG, so that you can remain healthy for many decades after your career is over.

LIVER AND ONIONS

(Libby Wade)

Organs are among the best suppliers of protein and iron. They contain amino acids that aid in digestion, bringing the nutrients into the body quickly. Liver and Onions is an old standby recipe, is easy to prepare, delicious, and is very inexpensive.

Ingredients:

6-8 oz. - Sliced liver (calves or beef)

1 medium onion

2 oz. – olive oil

2 pats – butter

1 tiny pinch - dried lavender

2 cloves – garlic

Salt and Pepper to taste

Dice onion and garlic, and slice liver into whatever size and shape you desire. Heat oil and 1 pat butter in pan and add garlic and onions. Sauté until onions are clear.

Add pinch of lavender and stir briefly then put in liver. Turn liver over several times, so that the juices are kept inside of it, and cook until the center is just past pink but not dry.

Remove liver and onions from pan. Turn heat to high, add pat of butter and salt and boil vigorously until sauce reduces. Pour this over liver and onions and eat.

VEGETARIAN CANNELLONI

(Ken Ludden)

This cannelloni recipe is fairly straight up to make, but it is a complex mixture of tastes. In the end, it is one of the most delicious tastes, and is great frozen and then heated in the microwave later. It is high in protein, carbohydrates and iron. The fact that it is a vegetarian recipe does not come from any lifestyle choice or political stance. It is vegetarian solely because it is filling, light and without the sort of aftermath that eating red meat gives. There is nothing worse in a training period than having a fatty protein hangover.

It can be made in bulk, reheated without losing any flavor, and serving size is very easy to determine. Cannelloni pasta has a bad reputation for being difficult to manage, particularly when it is being stuffed. Due to the nature of the filling in this recipe, however, that difficulty is overcome with a technique perfected for this very recipe. The only thing to be wary of with this recipe is that once you make it, others will constantly request it. And if you've made a batch and it is frozen, better put a lock on your freezer because if word gets out, it will be gone soon!

Pre-heat oven to 350°; and set out frozen chopped spinach to thaw so that it is room temperature when you are making the dish.

Ingredients:

2 boxes of cannelloni shells (12 per box, 24 total)

½ cup olive oil

Salt

Purified or filtered water

2 boxes frozen, chopped spinach

8 oz. Racotta cheese

8 oz. Fontina (grated or crumbled)

8 oz. Mozarella (grated)

3 cups grated Romano or Asiago cheese

16 oz. small curd cottage cheese

6 eggs

7 cloves garlic, finely minced

1 large onion, finely chopped

½ tsp anchovy paste

9 capers

2 tsp dill weed

½ tsp cayenne

½ tsp oregano

1 cup finely chopped Italian parsley

½ pint heavy whipping cream

Fill large boiling pot 2/3 full of purified or filtered water, pour in olive oil and 1 tblsp salt. Cover and set on high heat to boil.

When water is boiling, uncover and put cannelloni shells into water making sure they pass through the olive oil on the way in. Boil until very *al dente* (what would be considered 2/3 cooked).

Remove from boiling water by pouring through colander, and then run under cold water for 5 minutes. Remove from cold water and separate shells from each other on parchment. Let sit to cool.

In medium sized mixing bowl mix together Romano, Racotta, Fontina and Mozarella cheeses. Crumble with fingers after mixing to make sure they are evenly mixed and consistent in texture.

Remove 1/3 of mixture and set aside in smaller bowl.

Place minced garlic, capers and anchovy paste on cutting board and cut repeatedly with chopping knife so they are mixed evenly and capers are well cut up. Shake salt over this mixture until it looks like freshly fallen snow that has just begun to stick on road surface.

With the side of the chopping knife smash the garlic, caper, salt and anchovy paste mixture until it is a paste itself, and garlic pieces have turned clear and are broken down into liquid. Place in large mixing bowl.

Add eggs, oregano, dill, and cayenne to this mixture and beat until slightly frothy. Then add spinach, parsley and cottage cheese and stir thoroughly. When evenly mixed pour in 2/3 cheese mixture and ½ whipping cream and stir until evenly mixed.

Coat large baking dish with oil and place between cannelloni and filling. One at a time, take a cannelloni, split it so it is flat in your hand. Put enough of filling mixture to cover surface about ¾" and then return cannelloni to its cylindrical shape and place it seam down into baking dish. Do this, lining the stuffed cannelloni next to each other, tightly held in the breadth of the dish. Do this until the entire dish is filled with one layer of stuffed cannelloni.

> NOTE: Normally with this recipe it will take three or four baking dishes, depending on size.

Pour a thin layer of cream over the cannelloni, and then crumble 1/3 cheeses mix evenly over top and lightly salt. Bake for 1 hour, until top cheese is evenly melted and light brown on top of bubbles in it.

Serve hot or cold.

POLLO ALLA PRINCIPESSA

(Cici Mangioni di Palma)

While this recipe is very healthy, inexpensive, and quick to prepare, its greatest asset perhaps is that it is extremely impressive. When you are a dancer, student an professional, you often find yourself needing to host on the spur of the moment. And in the dance world, legendary and celebrity persons walk among the mortals all of the time. So many times when you must suddenly entertain, among your guests will be someone it serves well to impress. This recipe achieves this.

Always keep a couple of boneless, skinless chicken breasts in your freezer, some juniper berries and flat noodles in your cupboard, and a block of hard Romano or Asiago cheese in the fridge. Mushrooms and heavy cream you may have to get, but they are cheap and readily available in nearly any market.

Ingredients:

Olive oil

Butter

1 chicken breast (per person)

1 medium yellow onion

2 cloves garlic (1 per person and 1 for the
    pot)

½ cup sliced mushrooms (per person)

2 dried juniper berries (1 per person and 1
    for the pot)

1 pint heavy whipping cream (for 2 people,
    1 quart for 3-9 people)

Salt and Pepper (to taste)

Large, flat egg noodles

Dice onion and mince garlic, set aside.

Cut chicken breast(s) into cubes (approximately 1.5"-2") and set aside.

Fill pasta boiling pot with filtered water, add salt and float oil on top and bring to a simmer, then keep it at a simmer, covered.

Into a large, deep frying pan put olive oil and two pats butter and heat to slow sizzle. Sauté onions and garlic at low temperature until onions are clear. Turn up heat to medium and put in chicken cubes. Toss them constantly so that the outside surfaces are all cooked.

Throw in juniper berries and stir. Then pour whipping cream over top. Turn heat to high so that cream comes to rolling boil.

DO NOT TOUCH OR STIR!

Allow Chicken to boil vigorously, undisturbed for twelve minutes.

> NOTE: You will be tempted to stir this, as well anyone who walks by. Do not allow it to be touched. It will boil until greatly reduced in liquid volume. If it is stirred the cream will separate and the dish is utterly ruined!

Turn heat under pasta water to high, and when simmer becomes boil (almost instantly if it is simmering) put in noodles.

After 12 minutes, turn heat to medium and arrange mushrooms on top, completely covering the entire surface of the open pan.

DO NOT TOUCH OR STIR!

When mushrooms are dark and have sweat completely covering them, cover the whole mixture with finely grated Romano or Asiago cheese.

Using WOODEN SPOON gently fold chicken mixture, mushrooms and cheese just enough to basically mix it.

Drain noodles and place in pasta dish. Pour chicken mixture over top of noodles and present to table.

NOTE: Some people have trouble digesting juniper, so warn your guests of this fact and advise them to remove the juniper berries from their serving if they have received one on their plate. Because this dish requires a very hands-off approach so it doesn't fail, it is best to have guests remove the berries than to do it yourself prior to serving. However, if children are at table, then it is best to remove them yourself, or monitor their plates and do it there. They can cause a tummy ache in children easily.

This dish, served with an exotic salad, will be remembered by your guests. They will be convinced that you have a Haute Cuisine Chef hiding in your kitchen. This recipe is indeed a royal treasure.

PERFORMANCE RECIPES

Any performance requires freedom to focus on the task at hand without any distraction. It also requires the body to be energized and ready, without difficult digestive tasks that would inhibit your ability to give your full energetic attention to the task at hand.

During performance periods your nutritional intake must give you ample fuel to perform at peek capacities, and to provide adequate nutritional tools to rebuild any muscles that get over-stressed during the performance. The recipes in this section provide such foods. They are easy to digest, delicious, nutritious and quick enough to prepare that your time will not be needlessly spent in the kitchen.

PROPER PORRIDGE

(BQ)

BQ's "Proper Porridge", as she called it, has more to do with the method of preparation than the recipe itself. She was very opposed to quick oats, because she imagined that they create them by taking porridge and spreading it thin to dry, and then just breaking up the dried food into little bits. As humorous as this is, it is close to the truth. And the main objection is that they have previously been cooked, so they are not fresh and lacking in nutrients when you finally eat them.

Her use of a double-boiler is innovative and allows for the porridge to be set up the night before, so that in the morning all you must do is turn on the flame under the pot. By the time you emerge from your morning shower you have perfect porridge that is very delicious.

Ingredients:

2/3 Milk

1/3 water

1 pat Butter

¼ tsp. Salt

Rolled, Whole Oats

1 tblsp. Wheat Germ

The overall proportion of liquid to oats is 2:1, this is because oats expand to just under twice their dry size when cooked. Using rolled, whole oats (or just whole oats) gives the very best nutrients and is the most complete food with which to fuel your day of dance performance.

Fill the bottom of a double-boiler so that the water does not quite touch the bottom of the top container when put together.

Into the top container of the double-boiler put a mixture that is 2/3 milk and 1/3 water such that the total liquid is twice the amount of oats being cooked. Add ¼ tsp. of salt per serving to the liquids. Then stir in oats, and 1 tblsp. wheat germ and stir until salt is dissolved. Float butter pats on top. Cover and let sit for minimum 20 minutes.

When you are ready to eat, turn on stove flame to high and leave for 18 minutes. Turn off heat and take off lid. Stir and then serve.

This will give you creamy, delicious and nutritious Proper Porridge every time, and BQ will be pleased.

COLD TUNA (OR CHICKEN) ORZO SALAD

(Rita Ludden)

This dish was prepared by my mother when I had a run of performances and would be returning home after the rest of the family had eaten. It is delicious, keeps well, and invites eating one's fill without it bogging down the body.

Ingredients:

6 cups cooked orzo (chilled)

2 12 oz. tins of tuna, stored in water ; or equivalent of cooked, diced white chicken meat

1 cup mayonnaise

¼ cup chopped onions

2 cloves garlic minced

1 cucumber (remove skin and seeds and cut into ¼" cubes)

1 tsp Dijon mustard

Salt and Pepper to taste

Place all ingredients in mixing bowl and stir until evenly mixed. Serve on bed of lettuce, in hollowed tomato, or with sliced avocado.

Avocado, Lime, Hearts of Palm Salad

(Eric Darius)

This salad is absolutely delicious. Eric Darius, a friend, is also a sign language interpreter and has worked with many famous recording artists in concerts. This combination of tastes is his own invention and is so memorable.

> Ingredients:
>
> Baby Spinach
>
> Arugula
>
> Romaine
>
> 1 can hearts of palm cut into ¼" thick rounds
>
> 1 can Mandarin orange sections
>
> 2 avocados cut into ½" cubes
>
> Juice of one lime
>
> Chopped cilantro
>
> Balsamic vinegar
>
> Mini fresh mozzarella balls
>
> Salt and Pepper to taste

Place lettuces into salad bowl and mix. In the center place hearts of palm, Mandarin orange slices, avocado and mozzarella balls. Working from outside of the bowl and scooping from opposing sides down under and up through the center mix all ingredients.

After they are mixed, lightly sprinkle salt and pepper evenly across top, and then squeeze lime onto the salad.

> NOTE: Either wrap lime in cheese cloth to filter the pulp and seeds out, OR squeeze through a small hand-held strainer.

Using the cap of the Balsamic vinegar bottle, splash two caps full around the top of the salad, then toss and serve.

LIME AIOLI AND CRABMEAT

(Buenaventura, Tito's Chef and Assistant)

This dish was a favorite of Margot's, and whenever her husband's assistant (Buenaventura) traveled with her he prepared this for a light meal before performance.

Lime Aioli

Ingredients:

3 garlic cloves, finely minced

½ tsp. Dijon mustard

2 egg yokes

1/8 tsp salt

Juice of ½ lime

2 cups safflower oil

On cutting board, salt minced garlic and press into paste. Mix paste and mustard in copper mixing bowl. With weighted and balanced whisk, whip in egg yokes until smooth and creamy.

Continue to whip mixture while you dribble in the oil. Never add oil when mixture is not in vigorous movement, and with each dribbled addition of oil whip so that mixture remains as a solid of pudding consistency. Continue until all of the oil is mixed in and the mixture is a light yellow color.

Pour the filtered lime juice on top while mixture is still. Then whip until lime juice is completely mixed in and the color turns white.

Ingredients:

Water cress

Crab meat (drained if minced)

Paprikosch

Lime wedges

Take each plate, and cover it with water cress, and place a dollop of Lime Aioli in the center. Then place a ring of crab meat around this. Lightly sprinkle paprikosch on top of crab meat, place lime wedge into dollop of aioli, and then serve with fish fork.

Opening Night Tomato Soup

(George Jackson)

This recipe was put together one opening night after the show by Washington Post dance critic George Jackson. He whipped this up with ingredients he had in his pantry, and it was a perfect post-performance meal. Typically he barely remembered it when I served it back to him more than a decade later. It has become an opening night ritual for me.

Ingredients:

1 can of tomato soup concentrate

2 cups apple cider

½ cup white hominy (or ¼ cup dry grits)

Cracked black pepper

¼ cup chopped cilantro

Mix soup concentrate and apple cider in sauce pan and heat on low flame; stir until mixed. Add hominy, stir briefly and then cover and let simmer for 10 minutes.

Uncover and stir, pour into bowl, and float pepper on top with a sprinkling of chopped cilantro. Serve with interesting flat bread or cracker of complementary flavor.

Spaghetti Carbonare

(Cicci)

The beauty of this dish is that it can be prepared in as long as it takes to boil water and cook spaghetti. Cicci, who was our director for several productions, often whipped this up at opening night parties and post-performance meals. It is quick, nutritious and tastes great.

The dish itself comes from the Bologna region of northern Italy, and directly from the sheep and goat herders. By using dried meat, dried cheese, dried pasta, pepper corns, milk from the livestock, and fresh eggs, they were able to carry with them an entire meal that could last without refrigeration.

Ingredients:

Bacon – lean and cut into 1.5" sections

Eggs (one per person plus one for the pot)

Romano cheese – grated

Pepper Mill

Put on pasta water to boil (salt water and float oil on top). Fry bacon in pan. When pasta water boils put pasta in water. Beat eggs, adding 40 turns of the pepper mill. Grate cheese.

Drain pasta and put in pasta dish, pour eggs over top, crumble bacon and put on top, and pour bacon drippings onto mixture. Stir all ingredients except cheese together. The heat of the pasta and bacon oil will cook the eggs.

Add grated cheese so that noodles are evenly coated, and put the rest of the cheese on the table so people can season to taste.

TRAVEL RECIPES

Travel is a very major part of any dancer's career, and proper nutrition is even more important on the road because the body must adjust to changing climate, bedding, food and water. On tour the dancers have less time to prepare for performances because stage hands are preparing the stage far closer to performance time than in a home theater.

Dancers will often become injured on tour, both due to the grueling schedule and the constantly changing environment. And so the nutrition taken in must shield the dancers against potential injury, and be restorative for the muscles so that the continuous and minor daily stresses do not accumulate and become major problems.

Consistency of diet helps greatly, and without it dancers might suffer irregularity, and other gastro-intestinal discomfort. It is wise to begin a tour diet the week before tour begins.

TRAVELING CHEESE SANDWICHES

(Rita Ludden)

Traveling cheese sandwiches were a favorite on family trips when my siblings and I were young and we were on family vacations. They are easy to make, delicious and have plenty of protein and carbohydrates, as well as grain in the bread.

Ingredients:

1 cup grated cheddar cheese

2.5 tblsps. Mayonnaise

Sliced bread

Mix grated cheddar cheese with mayonnaise in bowl. Spread on bread and make into sandwiches.

NOTE: Different cheeses have different flavors and different amounts of salt. You may want to experiment as you mix this. There is also a wide variety of different sorts of mayonnaise and sandwich spreads. Invent the combination and proportions that taste the best to you.

Perky-Jerky

(Ken Ludden)

Little boosts of protein throughout the day are as important to the dancer as are carbohydrates. This is because each of these break down into glucose, the sugar that is the fuel all body processes comsume.

Beef Jerky was an early form of preservation of meat as a protein source. Since killing a large animal did not happen every day, and often many months would pass without having a source of meat, preserving it so it would not go bad was a way to keep people alive during winters, times of tribal migration or surviving in new surroundings that are not yet familiar. The technology developed by these early people serves dancers perfectly.

Jerky is nearly pure protein, and does not spoil. It is perfect for dancers to carry with them, and gives a protein boost. When dancers travel and do not have the option of familiar resources, nor the convenience of a kitchen or refrigerator, then having such foods will allow the body to receive the needed nutrition without the chance of a reaction to unfamiliar foods.

Pre-heat oven to 200°.

Ingredients:

4 pounds Beef, pork, lamb, veal, sheep, horse, duck, goose, venison—cut into ¼" thick strips

2 cups Olive oil

3 tblsps Pickling Spices

7 cloves garlic, minced

2 medium onions, finely chopped

2 cups red wine Vinegar

3 tblsps Worcestershire Sauce

2 tblsps Dijon Mustard

9 crushed capers

½ cup Mayonnaise

Seasonings

3 tblsps Salt

Place all ingredients except for meat into a large mixing bowl, and beat until smooth. Let sit for 2 hours.

Dip strips of meat into mixture, then place in large, deep baking dish, making sure that every strip of meat is completely covered with mixture. Cover with waxed paper and leave at room temperature for 4 hours, then refrigerate overnight.

Remove strips of meat, and skim off liquid mixture by passing them through your fingers. Place them on slightly oiled cookie sheets so that they are not overlapping.

Bake in oven for 3 hours, turn them over and bake another 3 hours. Turn off oven and leave overnight without opening oven door.

Remove from oven the next morning and pat them dry of oil with paper towel. Place them on drying racks sitting on paper towels, and leave them for another several hours.

> NOTE: Add seasonings to taste, depending on type of meat used. Be creative by adding flavors you enjoy, including such things as sesame oil, Vegemite, plum sauce, tomato juice, V8 juice, citrus, wine, beer, salad dressings, baby food fruit purees, Tabasco and other hot sauces, etc.

The resulting jerky will be very tasty and will last for a very long time. It is good to carry in a closed container in your dance bag (so that the smells don't get into your clothing), or in zip lock baggies for easy access throughout the day, or when traveling.

BLACK SESAME LAVASH

(Sallie Wilson)

There are many products that can be purchased when traveling that will constitute the nutritive mainstay of your dance diet. Such things as canned fish and meats, yogurts, soups, and dips (such as guacamole, humus, couscous, etc.) are readily available, and will have unique regional versions. There are many pickled and fermented foods as well that are consistent in quality and nutritive value that you will always be able to find, such as olives, pickles, pickled fruits and vegetables, sauerkraut, and more.

Added to these you will have fresh fruits and vegetables in each region, nutritive drinks, and dried sausages to fill out your travel diet. And there are always nuts and dried fruits as well.

The missing link is bread and other grain products. Granted, these are always available in every locale, but sometimes shops are closed when you are in the theater, or during the odd times in a dancer's day that it is possible to go out shopping, and you do want fresh bread.

Sallie Wilson, known as the greatest dramatic ballerina of the 20th century, had her favorites of canned, pickled, fermented and dried foods that she carried with her on tour. But the one thing she made herself was black sesame lavash. The recipe is easy to make, and very lightweight to carry with you on the road. Here is the recipe that evolved as she traveled in its final version.

Pre-heat oven to 275°

Prepare large flat cookie sheets by spraying with Olive Oil PAM, or rubbing with olive oil by hand.

Ingredients:

4 cups unbleached wheat flour

2 cups light rye flour

4 tsps salt

3 cups black sesame seeds

1 cup olive oil

1 cup water

4 eggs and two egg yokes (beaten)

White of two eggs

½ tsp. Vegemite

Cracked black pepper

Crushed Tibetan Pink Salt

Sift flours together well and put into large mixing bowl, and dig trough in center. In separate bowl, mix olive oil, water and beaten eggs. Whip until light froth forms. Add salt and black sesame seeds.

Pour liquid mixture into trough in center of dry mixture and stir the flour into the liquid in quick, progressive circular movements of the wooden spoon that gradually pull in the dry mixture.

When all of the flour is mixed in with the liquid, remove the spoon. Knead by hand until dough holds together in a ball, and a satin sheen forms on the surface.

In baseball-sized lumps, roll out the dough thin enough to almost be able to read through and place in cookie sheet, completely filling sheet to all of its edges.

Now mix the egg whites and Vegemite with just a tablespoon of water so that it is mixed evenly. Brush this mixture on entire top surface of the dough. Sprinkle cracked pepper and crushed Tibetan pink salt on top and spray lightly with olive oil PAM.

Bake for 2 hours, until edges are dark brown and least cooked part is golden brown.

Remove from oven and let cool for 1 hour. Then crash the pan onto the counter surface breaking the lavash into irregular pieces. Let sit over night, then package for travel in airtight containers.

This recipe will give you plenty of lavash. It is delicious with nearly any dip, and excellent with soups, broths, stew and other meals.

> NOTE: There was a period of time in which Sallie rolled out the lavash and cut it into neat 2" squares for baking. This made packaging it easier, but in

the end she reverted to the random mosaic that came from smashing it saying it was "more fun" to eat. However, this period came when Oliver Smith had told her she was no longer to be listed as a principal dancer with ABT, and I believe she needed to smash things at that point, so she returned to the original. But also, Sallie loved fun, so who knows?

CURRY PASTIES

BQ traveled all around the world, first as a young wife and mother, then later as the mother of the famous ballerina, Margot Fonteyn. She loved food and foreign cultures, and had developed a taste for some Asian and Oriental foods, though she stayed away from very spicy foods later in life as many must.

As a Londoner she enjoyed meat pies, which the British call "pasties". And when she learned about the Ludden Family "Never Fail Pie Crust" she got very excited about making her own pasties for a time. The first was a steak and kidney stew, which she put into the center of pastry dough to make snacks that I would carry with me to classes in London.

Then she decided that putting curry into these pasties would be excellent, which it was indeed, and by making the curry herself she could control the amount of spice in it.

To create these curry pasties, take any curry and let it cool to room temperature, or take from refrigerator and start with it cold.

Pre-heat oven to 350°. Prepare cookie sheet by putting parchment or waxed paper on the inside surface.

Make large batch of "Never Fail Pie Crust" recipe. Roll out to ¼ " thick. With rim of small bowl (Japanese bowls work very well for this as they are a perfect size and have a thin rim) and cut dough into rounds.

Place a teaspoon of curry to one side of the center line of the pastry round. Lifting the edge of the dough on the side that carries the curry dollop, fold over the curry so that the edge of the circle of dough is inside of the outer edge of the other side, making a half-moon shape.

Dampen the exposed edge with water and a brush (not too wet) and fold over the top edge, then roll the two together and pinch them into a decorative shape.

Pierce the center top of each pasty with a fork to let steam escape, and place evenly, with ¼" between on all sides, on baking sheet. Then bake for 35 minutes. Remove with pancake turner and place on drying rack and let fully cool. Leave out over night, (unless it is very hot and humid) before placing them in Tupperware container.

Store in layers with waxed paper between, and keep refrigerated until used. They will last at room temperature for about 3 days before going bad, but will last in refrigerator for up to one month.

They may be frozen, but sometimes if there is any moisture inside of the container, this will ruin the crust when thawed or heated.

DAY-OFF RECIPES

On days off it is important for dancers to enjoy themselves, and eat good food. It is important to enjoy and relax, but you cannot afford to put on extra weight in times of rest.

There is one recipe I made for days off that is delicious, nutritious and tastes very special indeed.

When I have a week off, I will make a large double batch of these and eat them throughout my time off.

RAISIN-NUT TARTS

(Ken Ludden)

Pre-heat oven to 350

Crust

Ingredients:

1 8-oz. package cream cheese

3 sticks margarine

3 cups flour

Put all ingredients in mixing bowl and let sit until room temperature. Mix by hand until it forms a single ball. Roll to 1/8" thick and cut circles with top of Japanese rice bowl. Place dough circles into muffin tin.

Filling

2 sticks margarine

3 cups sugar

6 egg yolks (save the whites for later)

2 teaspoons ground clove

1/4 teaspoon salt

6 tablespoons vinegar

2 teaspoons vanilla

2 lbs. raisins

2 lbs. chopped walnuts

6 egg whites, beaten until fluffy

Cut margarine and sugar until fluffy in a large bowl. Add egg yolks and stir until smooth. Add clove, salt, vinegar and vanilla, stir until color is consistent throughout. Stir in raisins and walnuts.

In a copper bowl, beat egg whites until fluffy but not dry. Fold egg whites into filling mixture. Spool filling into tarts. Bake until tops are dark golden brown (about 20 min).

Remove from oven (optional: sprinkle bourbon on tops while hot) and let cool for 1 hour before lifting tarts from muffin tins.

SICILIAN TOMATO SAUCE

(Hostess at Sicilian Soccer Summer Training)

In an active dancer's life there are few vacations. When vacations come, then, they must be enjoyed. One of my favorite memories was of a time when I had a Eurail pass and just traveled around. Due to train schedule problems in Italy I ended up meeting a young soccer player on his way to summer training in Sicily.

In our train cabin there was a woman and her family. She organized all of our food into a grand feast we all enjoyed during the trip. And when we got to Sicily she invited us to her house for dinner. At the dinner she made this recipe, which was the best tasting tomato sauce I had ever had, and remains so to this day. She gave me the recipe and I share it here with you.

Ingredients:

1 large white onion (finely diced)

½ cup olive oil

2 pats butter

1 lb. Italian sausage (mild or hot, per taste)

4 medium beefsteak tomatoes

6 bell tomatoes'

1 cup finely diced baby carrots

1 28 oz, can crushed tomatoes

6 cloves of garlic

7 capers

1 tsp anchovy paste

1 tsp salt

2 cups sliced mushrooms

1 tsp. ground, dried basil

½ tsp. celery salt

½ tsp. thyme

½ tsp. marjoram

½ tsp. powdered sage leaf

2 tsp. finely diced parsley

¼ tsp. oregano

½ tsp. cayenne

1 tsp. ground black pepper

Remove sausage meat from casing and form into 1.5" diameter balls. Set aside.

Sauté onion in skillet (medium heat) with ½ cup olive oil and two pats butter until onion is clear.

Add sausage balls and actively *sauté* at high heat until outside is evenly seared. Place mixture in large sauce pan, reduce heat to lowest and let simmer.

On cutting board, dice garlic cloves into very small pieces, along with capers. Form into hill in center of cutting board, put anchovy paste on top of hill, and dust evenly with salt. Using the flat side, blade edge, of a large kitchen chopping knife and smear until mixture forms an even, smooth paste. Put paste with simmering mixture and stir until evenly distributed, cover sauce pan.

Finely chop baby carrots in Cuisinart, then add to quartered tomatoes in large smoothie blender. Blend until an even *purée*. Pour over simmering mixture and increase flame to half heat. Open can of crushed tomatoes and add to the rest. Stir until fully mixed.

Bring to rolling boil while stirring, then reduce to active simmer. Add mushroom slices and herbs. Leave uncovered and simmering for 30 minutes.

Coat pasta noodles with olive oil, cook in brine until *al dente*. After draining noodles of brine, splash with thinnest liquid from sauce and carry to table.

Serve plates of pasta covered with sauce, and add finely grated, well-aged *Romano* cheese to individual taste.

GUACAMOLE

(Steven Capwell, 2nd President of Board)

Steven Capwell was the second president of the Summergate Dance Theater, Inc. board of directors. Under his direction we developed our Salon series into a major cultural event in the Washington, DC landscape, and mounted a world premier at the Kennedy Center.

At one of our Salons, he made this guacamole, and it instantly became a favorite. Every summer break this is a standard feature.

Ingredients:

3 Avocados

1 small lime

2 ripe tomatoes

1 onion

3 cloves garlic

3 capers

60 turns pepper

½ tsp cayenne

½ tsp salt

2 tbsp cilantro (dice finely – cut w/scissors)

Mash Avocado with lime juice. Dice onion, garlic, capers then blend with tomato until mush. Mix all other ingredients together with mush.

POISSON DIANNE

(Ken Ludden in honor of Libby Wade)

This recipe evolved during the years I had Libby Wade as my main dance partner. Her fiancé (later husband) David was a world traveler, and introduced many exotic flavors to our collective palate.

This recipe is one that was picked up during travels in Europe somewhere along the way. BQ had told me to always ask the Chef to order for me, and then request a recipe from the resultimg meal from the chef. She pointed out that whatever the recipe is you ask for, the Chef will tell you it is a secret, and then give you another one from the meal.

When I first tasted this, it was in a restaurant in Alsace. The fact that the gruyere cheese was fresh and had been made in that town made it all the more special. And upon returning from that trip and making it for Libby, it instantly became the second most requested recipe. It is brilliant, and it is always associated in memory as being for Libby. It has come to symbolize our years of dance partnership on stages around the world.

Pre-heat oven to 350°.

1 stick Butter

8 Tbsp White Flour

40 turns Pepper

1 Tbsp Salt

1 Tsp Dijon Mustard

1 Tsp Ground Nutmeg

4 cups Milk

1 lb + 1 cup Gruyere Cheese

White Fish

Seedless Green Grapes

Melt 1 stick of butter and 8 tablespoons white flower together in top part of a double boiler, right over the range. Stir until it is an even mixture and cook until it becomes golden brown.

Add 40 turns of the pepper mill, 1 tablespoon salt, 1 teaspoon Dijon mustard, and 1 teaspoon of ground nutmeg into the mixture. Have the bottom of the double boiler with 1.5" water already hot and put top pan over it. Using a whisk, add 4 cups milk slowly, and mix in so there are no lumps. Turn heat up to high and keep stirring in a figure-8.

When sauce starts to thicken sprinkle in 1 pound of grated Gruyere cheese and stir until melted.

Have filets of fish (flounder, or any salt water white fish) already covering the bottom of a greased baking dish (large square ones) and pour sauce over fish. Add another 1 cup of grated Gruyere cheese to top.

Bake at 350 degrees until cheese starts to brown. (20-40min). Serve hot with seedless green grapes cut in halves, chilled to almost frozen in freezer.

Enjoy!!!